NOURISHING ON A BUDGET

Cost-Effective Recipes for Prostate Cancer Wellness

DENNIS J. BELL

Copyright

All rights reserved. No part of this publication may reproduced, distributed or transmitted in any form or by any means including photocopying, recording or other electronic or mechanical method, without the prior written permission of the publisher, except in the case of brief quotation embodied in critical reviews and certain other non commercial uses permitted by copyright law.

Table of Contents

Chapter 1

Introduction to Prostate Cancer Nutrition

Prostate cancer is a common and serious disease affecting many men all over the world. It can cause a variety of symptoms and complications, including urinary problems, sexual dysfunction, bone pain, and metastasis (the spread of cancer to another organ). Prostate cancer treatment options include surgery, radiation therapy, hormone therapy, chemotherapy, or a combination of these. These treatments may also have side effects such as fatigue, nausea, loss of appetite, weight loss, and an increased risk of infection.

Nutrition has a significant impact on the outcome and quality of life of men with prostate cancer. A healthy diet can help prevent or manage some treatment side effects, boost the immune system, reduce inflammation, and lower the risk of disease recurrence or progression. Nutrition can also help you maintain a healthy body weight, which has been linked to higher survival rates and a lower risk of complications.

However, there is no one-size-fits-all diet for prostate cancer. Each man's nutritional requirements may differ depending on his age, stage of disease, treatment method, and other medical conditions. As a result, before making any dietary changes, it is recommended that you consult with a registered dietitian or healthcare provider. They can provide tailored advice and recommendations based on current scientific evidence and personal preferences.

Overview of the importance of nutrition during prostate cancer treatment

Nutrition is essential in helping the body cope with the stress and demands of prostate cancer treatment.

Some of the benefits of nutrition during prostate cancer treatment

• It can aid in the prevention or treatment of malnutrition, a condition in which the body lacks sufficient calories, protein, or other nutrients. Malnutrition can impair the immune system, increase the risk of infection, slow wound healing, and exacerbate treatment side effects. Malnutrition can also have a negative impact on men with prostate cancer's mental and emotional well-being, causing depression, anxiety, and low self-esteem.

• It can help with some of the most common treatment side effects, including nausea, vomiting, diarrhea, constipation, mouth sores, taste changes, and dry mouth. These side effects can make it difficult to consume enough food and water, leading to dehydration, weight loss, and nutrient deficiencies. A well-balanced diet rich in foods and fluids that are easy to digest, soothing, and appealing can help alleviate these symptoms while also increasing calorie and nutrient intake.

• It can help reduce inflammation, a process in which the immune system is activated to fight infections, injuries, or foreign substances. Inflammation is a natural and beneficial response that assists the body in healing and recovering. However, chronic or excessive inflammation can harm healthy cells and tissues, as well as contribute to cancer development and progression. Some dietary components, such as omega-3 fatty acids, antioxidants, and fiber, can help to regulate the inflammatory response and protect the body from oxidative stress and DNA damage.

• It can help reduce the risk of prostate cancer recurrence and progression. Certain dietary components, including saturated fat, red meat, processed meat, dairy products, and calcium, have been linked to an increased risk of developing or worsening prostate cancer. However, some dietary factors, such as lycopene, green tea, soy, vitamin D, and selenium, have been shown to have prostate cancer-preventing properties. A diet that limits or avoids harmful factors while increasing beneficial ones can help prevent or slow the growth and spread of prostate cancer cells.

Introduction to the concept of budget-friendly cooking for prostate health

Eating a healthy diet for prostate health does not have to be expensive or difficult. There are numerous ways to prepare delicious and nutritious meals that are both inexpensive and simple to make.

Some of the tips and strategies for budget-friendly cooking for prostate health

• **Plan ahead.** Planning your weekly meals and snacks can save you time, money, and energy. It can also help you avoid impulse purchases, food waste, and unhealthy lifestyle choices. You can find recipes that are appropriate for your taste, budget, and nutritional requirements using online tools, apps, or cookbooks. You can also check your local grocery store's sales and coupons to plan your meals around items that are on sale or in season.

• **Shop smart.** Shopping smart entails buying only what you need, getting the best deal, and properly storing and using your food.

Some of the ways to shop smart
• Make and stick to a shopping list. This can help you avoid purchasing unnecessary or unhealthy items that may tempt you at the store.
• Compare prices and quality between various brands and products. Look for the unit price, which indicates how much you will pay per ounce, pound, or other unit of measure. Choose the product with the lowest unit price while meeting your quality requirements.
• Purchase in bulk or in larger packages when possible. This can save you money per unit while also reducing packaging waste. However, ensure that you can consume or store the food before it spoils or expires.
• Buy fruits and vegetables that are frozen, canned, or dried. These products are typically

less expensive, last longer, and have comparable nutritional value to fresh produce. However, look for products that contain no added sugar, salt, or preservatives.

• Buy generic or store-brand products. These products are typically less expensive than name brands while maintaining the same quality and ingredients.

• Utilize coupons, discounts, or loyalty programmes. These can help you save money on certain items or earn rewards for making purchases. However, do not purchase items you do not need or want simply because they are on sale or have a coupon.

• Cook smart. Cooking smart entails using simple and healthy methods, ingredients, and equipment to prepare meals and snacks.

Some of the ways to cook smart

• Instead of frying, sautéing, or deep-frying, try low-fat cooking methods like baking, broiling, grilling, steaming, or microwaving. These methods can help you reduce the amount of fat and calories in your food while preserving its nutrients and flavor.

• Season your food with herbs, spices, lemon juice, vinegar, or salsa, rather than salt, butter, cream, cheese, or sauces. These can improve the flavor and aroma of your food while also providing antioxidants and other phytochemicals that may be beneficial to your prostate health.

• Use plant-based proteins such as beans, lentils, tofu, nuts, or seeds instead of or in addition to animal-based proteins like meat, poultry, fish, eggs, or dairy. Plant-based proteins are usually less expensive, have less fat and cholesterol, and contain more fiber and phytochemicals than animal-based proteins. They can also help you meet your protein requirements without exceeding your calorie intake.

• Make soups, stews, casseroles, salads, and smoothies from leftovers, scraps, or wilted produce. These can help you use up the food you already have and reduce food waste. These can help you use up the food you already have and reduce food waste.

Chapter 2

Budget-Friendly Breakfast Ideas

Breakfast is frequently referred to as the most important meal of the day because it provides the energy and nutrients required to start the day off right. Many people, however, skip breakfast or eat unhealthy foods like sugary cereals, pastries, or fast food due to a lack of time, money, or appetite. These choices can have a negative impact on the health and well-being of men with prostate cancer by increasing blood sugar levels, inflammation, and oxidative stress, while decreasing immune function and mood.

Simple and nutritious breakfast recipes using affordable ingredients

There are numerous inexpensive breakfast ideas that are both simple and nutritious, and can help promote prostate health without breaking the bank. These breakfast ideas are based on the following principles.

• Choose whole grains instead of refined grains. Whole grains, such as oats, quinoa, barley, and buckwheat, are high in fiber, antioxidants, and phytochemicals like lignans and phytosterols, which can help lower cholesterol, regulate blood sugar, and inhibit the growth and spread of prostate cancer cells. Refined grains, such as white bread, white rice, or white flour, are depleted of these beneficial components and can raise blood sugar levels and increase insulin resistance. Whole grains are also more filling and satisfying, which can help you avoid overeating and weight gain.

• Include a protein source in each breakfast. Protein is required for the growth and repair of muscles, tissues, and organs, as well as the production of hormones, enzymes and antibodies. Protein can also help men with prostate cancer control their appetites and maintain muscle mass, which is important because the disease or treatment can cause muscle loss.

However, not all proteins are equal. Some animal proteins, such as red meat, processed meat, and dairy products, can raise the risk of prostate cancer or worsen it because they contain saturated fat, cholesterol, hormones, or growth factors. Plant proteins, such as beans, lentils, tofu, nuts, or seeds, are preferable because they contain less fat and more fiber, as well as phytochemicals like isoflavones and saponins, which can modulate hormone levels, reduce inflammation, and induce apoptosis (cell death) in prostate cancer cells.

• Incorporate some fruits and vegetables into your breakfast. Fruits and vegetables are the richest sources of vitamins, minerals, antioxidants, and phytochemicals like carotenoids, flavonoids, and glucosinolates, which can protect cells from oxidative damage, boost the immune system, and prevent or slow the development and progression of prostate cancer.

Fruits and vegetables can also enhance the color, flavor, and texture of your breakfast, making it more appealing and enjoyable. Tomatoes, watermelon, pink grapefruit, carrots, pumpkin, broccoli, cauliflower, cabbage, Brussels sprouts, kale, and spinach are among the fruits and vegetables that are particularly good for prostate health.

Tips for preparing balanced breakfasts that promote prostate health without breaking the bank.

Here are some examples of budget-friendly breakfast recipes:

- **Oatmeal with berries and nuts**.

Oatmeal is a classic breakfast that is simple to prepare, inexpensive, and versatile. It can be cooked with water or plant-based milk, such as soy milk, almond milk, or oat milk, and sweetened with honey, maple syrup, or stevia. You can also add cinnamon, nutmeg, or vanilla extract to enhance flavor. Then, top it with fresh or frozen berries like blueberries, raspberries, strawberries, or blackberries, as well as chopped nuts like walnuts, almonds, or pistachios. Berries are high in anthocyanins, which are potent antioxidants that can protect against DNA damage and inflammation that can lead to prostate cancer. Nuts are high in omega-3 fatty acids, which are anti-inflammatory and can inhibit angiogenesis (the formation of new blood vessels that fuel tumor growth). This breakfast is high in fiber, protein, and healthy fats, and it will keep you satisfied and energized for hours.

- **Quinoa and vegetable scramble.**

Quinoa is a gluten-free grain high in protein, fiber, and minerals such as iron, magnesium, and zinc. It has a nutty flavor and a fluffy texture, making it an excellent substitute for rice and couscous. To prepare this breakfast, cook the quinoa according to package directions and set aside. In a skillet, heat olive oil and sauté chopped onion, garlic, bell pepper, mushroom, and spinach until soft and wilted. Season with salt, pepper, cumin, and turmeric. Turmeric is a spice rich in curcumin, a powerful anti-inflammatory and anti-cancer agent that can inhibit the proliferation and invasion of prostate cancer cells. Then, add the crumbled or cubed tofu and cook until browned. Tofu is a soy product high in protein and isoflavones, which can regulate estrogen and testosterone levels while inhibiting the growth and spread of prostate cancer cells. Finally, combine the quinoa and vegetable mixture, and serve with salsa or avocado. This breakfast is high in protein, fiber, and phytochemicals, making it a savory and satisfying way to start the day.

• **Banana and peanut butter smoothie.**
Smoothies are an excellent way to get a lot of nutrients in a liquid form, which can be especially beneficial for men with prostate cancer who have difficulty swallowing, chewing, or digesting solid foods. To make this smoothie, combine one ripe banana, one cup plant-based milk, two tablespoons peanut butter, one tablespoon flaxseed, and ice cubes. Banana contains potassium, which helps regulate blood pressure and fluid balance. Peanut butter is high

in protein and healthy fats, and it can enhance the smoothie's creaminess and sweetness. Flaxseed contains omega-3 fatty acids and lignans, which can help lower cholesterol, reduce inflammation, and prevent prostate cancer cells from growing and spreading. This smoothie is high in calories, protein, and healthy fats, which can help you meet your energy and nutritional requirements.

Chapter 3

Lunchtime Solutions: Soups, Salads, and Sandwiches

Lunch is an important meal because it allows you to refuel your body and mind while also providing the nutrients and energy you need to get through the rest of the day. However, many people have difficulty finding healthy and affordable lunch options, particularly when they are busy, on the go, or have limited access to a kitchen. This can lead to skipping lunch, eating out, or consuming processed or fast foods, all of which can have a negative impact on the health and well-being of men with prostate cancer by increasing their intake of calories, fat, sodium, sugar, and additives while decreasing their intake of fiber, antioxidants, and phytochemicals.

Budget-friendly lunch recipes that focus on cancer-fighting ingredients

Fortunately, there are numerous lunchtime options that are inexpensive, simple to prepare, and focus on cancer-fighting nutrients.

These lunchtime solutions are based on the following principles:

• Choose soups, salads, and sandwiches as your main lunch options. Soups, salads, and sandwiches are adaptable, simple, and fulfilling meals that may be prepared ahead of time, refrigerated or frozen, then warmed or assembled as needed. They can also be tailored to your preferences, budget, and nutritional requirements, and they can contain a number of components that promote prostate health. Soups, salads, and sandwiches are particularly good for staying hydrated since they include a lot of water and fluids, which help flush out toxins, avoid dehydration, and lower the risk of urinary tract infections.

• Use whole grains, beans, and vegetables as the base of your soups, salads, and sandwiches. Whole grains, beans, and vegetables are high in fiber, antioxidants, and phytochemicals including lignans, phytosterols, and glucosinolates, which can help lower cholesterol, manage blood sugar levels, and prevent the growth and spread of prostate cancer cells. They can also help you feel full and satisfied while preventing overeating and weight gain. Whole grains include brown rice, quinoa, barley, and whole wheat bread. Beans can include black beans, kidney beans, chickpeas, or lentils. Vegetables include things like tomatoes, carrots, broccoli, cabbage, and spinach.

• Add lean protein to soups, salads, and sandwiches. Lean protein is necessary for the development and repair of muscles, tissues, and organs, as well as the production of hormones, enzymes and antibodies. Lean protein can also help men with prostate cancer control their appetites and retain muscle mass, which is vital because the disease or therapy might cause muscle loss.

However, not all proteins are equal. Some animal proteins, such as red meat, processed meat, and dairy products, can raise the risk of prostate cancer or aggravate it because they include saturated fat, cholesterol, hormones, or growth factors. Plant proteins, such as tofu, tempeh, nuts, or seeds, are preferable because they are low in fat and high in fiber, as well as phytochemicals like isoflavones and saponins, which can adjust hormone levels, reduce inflammation, and promote apoptosis (cell death) in prostate cancer cells. Lean proteins include chicken breast, turkey breast, fish, eggs, and low-fat cheese.

• Dress up your soups, salads, and sandwiches with healthy fats, herbs, and spices. Healthy fats, such as olive oil, avocado, and nuts, can aid in the absorption of fat-soluble vitamins and antioxidants while also providing anti-inflammatory and anti-cancer properties.

Herbs and spices like garlic, ginger, turmeric, or basil can improve the flavor and aroma of your food while also providing antioxidants and phytochemicals like allicin, gingerol, curcumin, or eugenol, which can protect cells from oxidative damage, boost the immune system, and prevent or slow the development and progression of prostate cancer. However, avoid adding excessive amounts of salt, butter, cream, cheese, or sauces, since these can add calories, fat, sodium, and additives, increasing the risk of high blood pressure, heart disease, and kidney problems.

Here are some examples of budget-friendly lunch recipes that follow these principles:

- **Tomato and lentil soup.**

Tomato and lentil soup is a hearty and nutritious soup that is simple to prepare, inexpensive, and tasty. You can prepare it by sautéing chopped onion, garlic, celery, and carrot in olive oil until tender and fragrant. Then, add some vegetable broth, canned tomatoes, dried lentils, bay leaf, salt, pepper, and thyme, and bring to a boil.

Reduce the heat and cook until the lentils are cooked, which should take around 20 to 30 minutes. If you want to make the soup creamier, you can blend some of it. Tomato and lentil soup is packed in fiber, protein, and lycopene, a powerful antioxidant that can protect against DNA damage and inflammation, which can contribute to prostate cancer.

• **Chicken and spinach salad.**
Chicken and spinach salad is a light and refreshing salad that is simple to prepare, inexpensive, and delicious. To make it, combine some baby spinach leaves, sliced chicken breast, cherry tomatoes, cucumber, red onion, and feta cheese in a large bowl. Toss the salad with olive oil, lemon juice, salt, pepper, and oregano until completely combined. Chicken and spinach salad is abundant in protein, iron, vitamin C, and carotenoids, which are antioxidants that protect cells from oxidative damage, boost the immune system, and prevent or slow the spread of prostate cancer.

• **Turkey and avocado sandwich.**

Turkey and avocado sandwich is a simple yet delicious sandwich that is quick to prepare, inexpensive, and filling. Make it by spreading mashed avocado, mustard, and mayonnaise on two slices of whole wheat bread. Then, put some sliced turkey breast, lettuce, tomato, and cheese on one slice of bread and top with the other. Cut in half and enjoy.

Chapter 4

Dinner Delights on a Dime

Dinner is an important meal that may help you end your day on a happy note while also providing the nutrients and energy your body requires to recuperate and repair. However, many individuals find it difficult to prepare healthy and delicious dinners that are also cost-effective, particularly when they have limited time, money, or resources. This can lead to men with prostate cancer ordering takeout, eating processed or frozen foods, or skipping dinner entirely, all of which can have a negative impact on their health and well-being by increasing their intake of calories, fat, sodium, sugar, and additives while decreasing their intake of fiber, antioxidants, and phytochemicals.

Hearty and satisfying dinner recipes that are both affordable and nutritious

There are numerous evening pleasures that are both inexpensive and nutritious, and can benefit prostate health without costing a fortune.

These dinner delights are based on the following principles:

• Choose plant-based or lean animal proteins as the main component of your dinner. Plant-based proteins, such as beans, lentils, tofu, tempeh, nuts, and seeds, are high in protein, fiber, and phytochemicals like isoflavones and saponins, which can modify hormone levels, reduce inflammation, and cause apoptosis (cell death) in prostate cancer cells. They are also low in fat and cholesterol, and less expensive than most animal proteins. Lean animal proteins, such as chicken, turkey, fish, and eggs, are high in protein, iron, zinc, and selenium, all of which are necessary for the immune system, red blood cell synthesis, and antioxidant protection. They are also low in saturated fat and cholesterol and can be purchased in bulk or on sale for a discount.

However, avoid or limit red meat, processed meat, and dairy products since they include saturated fat, cholesterol, hormones, or growth factors, which might raise the risk of prostate cancer or worsen it.

• Use whole grains, beans, and veggies as the foundation or side dishes for your entrée. Whole grains, legumes, and vegetables are high in fiber, antioxidants, and phytochemicals including lignans, phytosterols, and glucosinolates, which can help lower cholesterol, manage blood sugar levels, and prevent the growth and spread of prostate cancer cells. They can also help you feel full and satisfied while preventing overeating and weight gain. Whole grains include brown rice, quinoa, barley, and whole wheat pasta. Whole grains include brown rice, quinoa, barley, and whole wheat pasta. Examples of veggies include tomatoes, carrots, broccoli, cabbage, and spinach.

• Season your dinner with healthy fats, herbs, and spices. Healthy fats, such as olive oil, avocado, and nuts, can aid in the absorption of fat-soluble vitamins and antioxidants while also providing anti-inflammatory and anti-cancer properties. Herbs and spices like garlic, ginger, turmeric, or basil can improve the flavor and aroma of your food while also providing antioxidants and phytochemicals like allicin, gingerol, curcumin, or eugenol, which can protect cells from oxidative damage, boost the immune system, and prevent or slow the development and progression of prostate cancer. However, avoid adding excessive amounts of salt, butter, cream, cheese, or sauces, since these can add calories, fat, sodium, and additives, increasing the risk of high blood pressure, heart disease, and kidney problems.

Here are some examples of dinner delights that follow these principles
- **Black bean and vegetable chili.**

Black bean and vegetable chili is a warm and satisfying dinner that is simple to prepare, inexpensive, and flavorful. Black bean and vegetable chili is a warm and satisfying dinner that is simple to prepare, inexpensive, and flavorful. Then, bring to a boil with vegetable broth, canned black beans, canned tomatoes, corn, salt, pepper, chili powder, cumin, and oregano. Reduce the heat and allow to simmer for 15 to 20 minutes, or until the flavors are fully blended. For added flavor, try adding chopped jalapeño, cilantro, or lime juice. Black bean and vegetable chili is strong in fiber, protein, and lycopene, a potent antioxidant that can protect against DNA damage and inflammation that can lead to prostate cancer.

• **Salmon and quinoa salad.**
Salmon and quinoa salad is a light and refreshing meal that is simple to prepare, inexpensive, and fulfilling. You can make it by cooking and fluffing quinoa according to package directions. Then, season some salmon fillets with salt, pepper, and lemon juice before baking for 15 to 20 minutes. In a large mixing bowl, combine baby spinach leaves, cherry tomatoes, cucumber, red onion, and feta cheese with olive oil, lemon juice, salt, pepper, and dill.

Then, flake the salmon and toss it into the salad with the quinoa until well combined. Salmon and quinoa salad is abundant in protein, omega-3 fatty acids, and vitamin E, all of which are anti-inflammatory and anti-cancer agents capable of inhibiting the proliferation and invasion of prostate cancer cells.

• **Chicken and broccoli stir-fry.**

Chicken and broccoli stir-fry is a simple yet tasty recipe that is quick to prepare, inexpensive, and filling. You can create it by slicing chicken breast into thin slices and marinating them in soy sauce, rice vinegar, honey, cornstarch, and ginger for 15 to 20 minutes. Then, in a large skillet over high heat, heat the sesame oil and stir-fry the chicken for about 10 to 15 minutes, or until browned and cooked through. Place the chicken on a plate and keep heated. In the same skillet, heat some more sesame oil and stir-fry some minced garlic, broccoli florets, and red pepper flakes until crisp-tender, about 5 to 10 minutes. Then add the chicken and the remaining marinade, and bring to a boil. Chicken and broccoli stir-fry has a lot of protein, iron, and glucosinolates, which are phytochemicals that can trigger detoxification and apoptosis in prostate cancer cells.

Chapter 5

Smart Snacking and Dessert Alternatives

Snacking and dessert are frequently regarded as luxuries that can derail a healthy diet, particularly among men with prostate cancer who must limit their consumption of calories, fat, sugar, and additives. Snacking and dessert can, however, be part of a balanced and nutritious diet if chosen thoughtfully and taken in moderation. Snacking and dessert can help men with prostate cancer satisfy their appetite and cravings while also providing energy and nutrients and improving their mood and well-being. However, not all snacks and desserts are made equal. Some snacks and desserts, such as chips, cookies, candy, or ice cream, are rich in calories, fat, sugar, and additives while poor in fiber, antioxidants, and phytochemicals.

These snacks and desserts can have a negative impact on the health and well-being of men with prostate cancer by increasing blood sugar levels, inflammation, and oxidative stress, while decreasing immune function and mood.

Quick and budget-friendly snack ideas to curb cravings and support prostate wellness

Fortunately, there are numerous smart snacking and dessert options that are quick and inexpensive, and can promote prostate health without sacrificing taste or enjoyment.

These snacking and dessert alternatives are based on the following principles:
• Choose snacks and sweets high in fiber, protein, and healthy fats, but low in sugar and additives. Fiber, protein, and healthy fats can help you feel full and satisfied while preventing overeating and weight gain. They can also help to manage blood sugar levels, reduce inflammation, and stop the growth and spread of prostate cancer cells. Sugar and additives can raise blood sugar levels, promote inflammation and oxidative stress, and impair immunological function and mood. Fresh or dried fruits, nuts,

seeds, granola bars, yogurt, hummus, popcorn, or dark chocolate are all examples of snacks and sweets that are high in fiber, protein, and healthy fats while low in sugar and chemicals.

• Opt for natural sweeteners like honey, maple syrup, or stevia instead than refined sugar, artificial sweeteners, or corn syrup. Natural sweeteners are less processed and contain vitamins, minerals, antioxidants, and phytochemicals that help improve the health and well-being of prostate cancer patients. Refined sugar, artificial sweeteners, and corn syrup are highly processed and contain no nutrients. They can have a negative impact on the health and well-being of men with prostate cancer by increasing blood sugar levels, inflammation, and oxidative stress while decreasing immune function and mood. However, use natural sweeteners carefully because they still have calories and can influence blood sugar levels.

• Opt for plant-based or low-fat dairy products like soy milk, almond milk, oat milk, or low-fat yogurt over full-fat dairy products like whole milk, cream, cheese, or ice cream. Plant-based or low-fat dairy products include less fat and cholesterol and more fiber and phytochemicals, such as isoflavones and saponins, which can regulate hormone levels, reduce inflammation, and cause apoptosis (cell death) in prostate cancer cells. Full-fat dairy products are higher in fat and cholesterol, and they contain hormones and growth factors that can increase the risk of prostate cancer or aggravate it.

Here are some examples of smart snacking and dessert alternatives that follow these principles:
• **Apple and peanut butter.**
Apple and peanut butter is a simple and delicious snack that is easy to prepare, inexpensive, and healthful. To make it, slice an apple and apply peanut butter on each piece. Apple contains fiber, vitamin C, and quercetin, an antioxidant that can protect cells from oxidative damage, boost the immune system, and prevent or halt the spread of prostate cancer. Peanut butter provides protein and healthy fats

while also adding creaminess and sweetness to the snack. This snack is high in fiber, protein, and healthy fats, and can keep you full and energized for hours.

- **Banana and oat muffins.**

Banana and oat muffins are a sweet and fluffy dessert that is simple to make, inexpensive, and delicious. Make these by mashing ripe bananas and combining them with eggs, honey, vanilla extract, and olive oil. Stir in some whole wheat flour, baking soda, salt, cinnamon, and oats until well combined. Spoon the batter into a muffin tin and bake for 15 to 20 minutes, until golden and cooked through. Banana and oat muffins are packed in fiber, protein, and potassium, which can aid with blood pressure and fluid balance. They are also naturally sweetened with honey and banana, with no refined sugars or chemicals. This dessert is full in fiber, protein, and potassium, so you can satisfy your sweet appetite guilt-free.

- **Berry and yogurt parfait.**

Berry and yogurt parfait is a colorful and refreshing treat that is simple to prepare, inexpensive, and tasty. In a glass or bowl, combine low-fat yogurt, fresh or frozen berries, and granola. If desired, you can drizzle the parfait with honey or maple syrup. If desired, you can drizzle the parfait with honey or maple syrup. It is also low in fat and sugar and free of additives. This dessert is high in protein, calcium, and antioxidants, and it will deliver a refreshing and creamy pleasure for your taste buds.

Conclusion

Prostate cancer is a frequent and deadly disease that affects millions of men worldwide. It can result in a variety of symptoms and complications, including urinary issues, sexual dysfunction, bone pain, and metastasis. Prostate cancer treatment options include surgery, radiation therapy, hormone therapy, chemotherapy, or a combination of these. These medications can also cause fatigue, nausea, loss of appetite, weight loss, and an increased risk of infection.

Nutrition has a significant impact on the outcome and quality of life of men with prostate cancer. A balanced diet can help prevent or manage some therapeutic side effects, boost the immune system, reduce inflammation, and lessen the risk of illness recurrence or progression. Nutrition can also help you maintain a healthy body weight, which has been linked to higher survival rates and a lower risk of problems.However, maintaining a good diet for prostate health does not have to be costly or difficult. There are numerous ways to cook delicious and nutritious meals that are both inexpensive and simple to make. By following the advice and practices in this book, you may nurture your body and mind, enhance your health and well-being, and save money and time. You can also enjoy more variety and flavor in your meals, making them more enticing and pleasurable.